Possibilities

that are YOU!

Volume 4: Conscious Compassion

by
Alex Bennet

D1516201

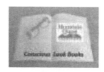

An imprint of **MQIPress** (2018)

Frost, West Virginia

ISBN 978-1-949829-06-8

MQIPress

Frost, West Virginia
303 Mountain Quest Lane, Marlinton, WV 24954
United States of America
Telephone: 304-799-7267
eMail: alex@mountainquestinstitute.com
www.mountainquestinstitute.com
www.mountainquestinn.com
www.MQIPress.com
www.Myst-Art.com

ISBN 978-1-949829-06-8
Verse by poet Cindy Lee Scott
Photos by Alex Bennet
Graphics by Fleur Flohil

Perceiving a glow about the face
Reaching outward with imparted grace
Teaching with chosen conscious action
Exuding loving warm compassion

Listening with a heart of silence
Receiving and open to guidance
Feeling the pulse of humanity
Giving forward, acting selflessly

Hungering for agápē perfection
Opening in the Love Soul Connection

-Cindy Lee Scott

Preface

This book is for YOU. Regardless of economic success or educational prowess, beyond cultural influences and habitual routines, YOU have been and continue to be a student of life. And since our time in this learning sphere is precious, the challenges and opportunities are both rapid and continuous, always offering new insights. YOU are a verb, not a noun. Forget what you were taught in grammar school!

Now, we live in a world of demanding challenges, where people and systems are rebounding from control, rebelling from eras of real and perceived suppression of thought. With the acceleration of mental development over the past century has come increased awareness of human capacity, with economic success in small bites for many and large bites for the few, and for some coming with an arrogance that says, "Look at me. I'm right, you're wrong, and I'm not listening."

Because of our Economy's focus on the material, economic success begets economic success and the separation of wealth grows larger, flaming the difficulties of surviving in a CUCA world, that is, a world of accelerating change, rising uncertainty, increasing complexity, and the anxiety that comes with these phenomena.

Yet all of this **offers us, as a humanity the opportunity to make a giant leap forward.** By opening ourselves to ourselves, we are able to fully explore who we are. With that exploration comes glimmers of hope as we contemplate the power of each and every mind developed by the lived human experience!

As YOU move through your life of thoughts, feelings and actions—even when you have to repeat things over and over again as part of the experience—YOU are advancing toward the next level of consciousness.

Here's the bottom line. Everything that has been learned and continues to be learned is out there … and as a student of life, YOU have access to it all. So often it is expressed in ways that don't make sense because of the language and media being used. It just isn't presented conversationally, and you don't have a chance to ask questions from your unique point of view.

So, these little books—which we refer to as Conscious Look Books—are specifically focused on sharing key concepts from *The Profundity and Bifurcation of Change* series and **looking at what those concepts mean to YOU**.

These books are conversational in nature, and further conversations are welcome. We invite your thoughts and questions, not guaranteeing answers because there is still so much to learn, but happy to

join in the conversation. Visit Mountain Quest Inn
and Retreat Center www.mountainquestinn.com
located in the Allegheny Mountains of West Virginia
or email alex@mountainquestinstitute.com

As my partner David reminds us: *Run with the future!*

Our gratitude to all those who take this journey with us, and a special thanks to the colleagues, partners, friends, family and visitors who touch our hearts and Mountain Quest in so many ways.

With Love and Light, Alex and David

Contents

Introduction (Page 1)

Idea 1: Developing compassion is part of our human developmental journey. (Page 5)

Idea 2: These times call for a Global Ethic. (Page 13)

Exercise: Tapping into a Universal Spirituality

Idea 3: Empathy developed while co-evolving is a stepping stone toward conscious compassion. (Page 19)

Idea 4: The act of judging can derail compassion. (Page 25)

Exercise: Discerning Judging

Idea 5: Compassion cannot be achieved when we retain strong negative emotions. (Page 33)

Idea 6: Conscious compassion is an intelligent choice to give selfless service. (Page 35)

Idea 7: Compassion is part of the larger journey toward unconditional love. (Page 47)

What does this mean to me? (Page 53)

Introduction

Compassion leads to, and is a companion of, unconditional love as the highest virtue of the emotional field. As we explore the virtue of compassion, we explore the depth of our growing connections with others, which is reflective in all of our life experiences.

People are complex systems made up of physical, mental, emotional and spiritual elements, and, fortunately for us, most of the time all of these elements are functioning. It is when we try to close one of them off that we get into trouble!

Going to one of my favorite dictionaries for help, the *American Heritage Dictionary* considers emotions as a spontaneous mental state and goes so far as to describe them as a feeling.[1] It's fascinating thinking about emotions as a mental state, although we do know, of course, that when we are emotional what we think of as our mental state is a bit fuzzy! When we're experiencing strong emotions, it's hard to think clearly and, well, logically.

Antonio Damasio—a neuroscientist, psychologist and philosopher, so he certainly ought to have some expertise in this subject—says there is a difference between emotions and feelings.[2] I tend to agree with him. After all, words are what we make of them.

It is convenient to think about emotions and feelings as different. Emotions are a collection of responses which are, most often, visible. When we look at or listen to someone who is angry, we know they are angry. Similarly, laughing and tears certainly clearly convey emotional states!

Antonio says that he reserves the term "feelings" for the private mental experience of emotion, something that is *felt* by the individual but not publicly observable. I guess we could say that emotions are externally focused, and feelings are internally focused.

With this understanding, let's explore the word itself. The "passion" part of compassion could certainly be considered both an emotion *and* a feeling, although when I'm passionate about something it generally comes through in my actions! So, what would "compassion" be? Hmmm. It's certainly a strong feeling of sympathy or empathy with a desire to help. Sympathy and empathy are explored later in this book.

Through words of kindness and caring we can *show* compassion, although this can be done in many ways; for example, through our actions and perhaps the tone of our voice. This may certainly occur in response to a specific event or situation—which is what happens through emotions—only *is it an emotional response or a conscious mental response?* All this gets quite confusing since at least two experts (Antonio and whoever wrote the dictionary definition) agree that emotions are a *mental state*.

In the big book, *The Profundity and Bifurcation of Change*, the idea of "cognitive conveyors" is introduced. This is a pretty interesting description of words that are filled with a combination of thought, emotion and feelings, and, while emotional arousal (emotions) play an important role both affecting mental activity and having a physiological effect on the body, these words are not identified specifically as emotions. Examples are desire, courage, drive and, just maybe, compassion.

For the conversation we are having now, let's think of compassion as both a cognitive conveyor *and* an inward feeling. Then, based on this inward feeling, if we choose, we *show* compassion through our words and actions.

This adds an interesting dimension to the feeling that goes along with compassion. *We have a desire to act on that feeling!* The prefix "com," which is part of compassion, conveys the meaning of together or with, so compassion literally means "with passion." That concept begs an object of passion, that we do something "with passion." Although, since this is a mental state, even the choice of *choosing not to act* would be an action!

The importance of this idea of conscious compassion, choosing to be compassionate, has been forwarded before by various participants in the school of life. For example, Michael Lerner, who interweaves a passion for politics and spiritual teaching, calls for each of us to put "conscious energy into developing a compassionate attitude toward all of being, all animals, and all human beings, including yourself."[3]

This higher order of compassion is what is meant by conscious compassion. It is the ability to recognize our internal feelings of compassion and, with morality and good character, choose our actions wisely.

Let's explore this further.

Idea 1: Developing compassion is part of our human developmental journey.

The Intelligent Social Change Journey, what we will refer to as the ISCJ, is a developmental journey of the body, mind and heart. As we expand and grow, we move from the heaviness of cause-and-effect linear extrapolations, to the fluidity of co-evolving with our environment, to the lightness of breathing our thought and feelings into reality.

Grounded in development of our mental faculties, these are phase changes, each building on and expanding previous learning in our movement toward intelligent activity.[4] Yet, we are on this journey together, so this is very much a *social* journey. Growth does not occur in isolation! The deeper our understanding in relationship to others, the easier it is to move into the future.

As we navigate the linear, cause-and-effect characteristics of Phase 1 of this journey, *the quality of sympathy* is needed. Then, *the quality of empathy* is required to navigate the co-evolving liquidity of Phase 2. And, as we move into Phase 3, *the quality of compassion* is needed to navigate the connected breath of the creative leap. I'll insert a figure of how that looks.

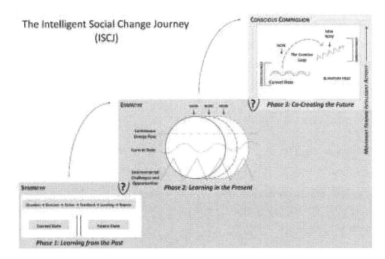

Figure 1. *The three phases of the ISCJ.*

That was a pretty quick description, sort of what we might call an overview. And, while it is all very interesting, how does it exactly relate to my personal journey?

Okay. Let's talk about that. In **Phase 1 of the ISCJ**, we learn from the past, remembering the responses to events that have happened in our lives. When we respond to events, we "see" the changes that happen with our eyes, and *therefore they are real*. Causes have effects and actions have consequences, both directly and indirectly, although sometimes delayed. For example, when we study for a test, we get a better grade. If we break the law, well, we hope there are consequences of some nature!

This first phase of living reinforces the characteristics of how we interact with the simplest aspects of our world. Responses to our actions become predictable and repeatable and make us feel comfortable because we know what to expect and how to prepare for them. While these things are certainly part of our experience, our brain tends to automate the thinking around them, and we do them with little conscious effort.

This linear cause-and-effect phase of the ISCJ *calls for sympathy*. It is a lot easier to navigate through relationships with a little bit of sympathy, and we can't exactly live without having relationships with other people! How about a work situation as an example? Let's say you have a disagreement with a colleague at work, and you know he's definitely wrong. So, not thinking, you dismiss his ideas, then turn to his boss (who is standing nearby) and tell him how it should be done.

Quite confident in your opinion, as you turn to leave you see your "former friend" standing behind you with his mouth still opened in amazement and surprise. As *his* boss pats *you* on the shoulder and walks away, ignoring your colleague, you realize what has just occurred. Did you really just do that? But "I'm right," you think, as your colleague turns away in anger and pain.

How do *you* feel? Are you sympathetic to your colleague's feelings? You might think about how you would feel if a "colleague and friend" had done that to you. How *would* you feel? Remember, others were there watching this event. Whatever relationship you had developed in the past with your colleague, and with your organization, is now in a state of flux.

Cause-and-effect events only remain predictable if all the causes that influence them remain constant. And that just doesn't happen in the world of today! While no doubt there are underlying beliefs or fears that drive our behaviors, our responses to situations can surprise even us. Eventually, over time, we begin to recognize patterns in different types of behaviors, and, if we choose to do so, begin to work on changing the behaviors that make us feel bad.

Expanding to **Phase 2 of the ISCJ**, we begin to recognize more and more patterns emerging from the events of life. *Recognition of patterns* enables us to "see" in our mind's eye. Through this process we *see* the relationship of events in terms of time and space, moving us out of an action-reaction mode into a position of co-evolving with our environment. This enables us to better navigate a world full of diverse challenges and opportunities.

<<<<<<<◇>>>>>>>

INSIGHT: **Recognition of patterns enables us to "see" in our mind's eye.**

<<<<<<<◇>>>>>>>

It is at this stage that we move from understanding based on *past* cause-and-effect reactions to produce new things both in the moment at hand and at a future point in time. This is a higher level of thinking and feeling about how we interact with our world, including the interesting area of human social interactions.

Although they may be complex, the patterns that we begin to recognize allow us to explore and progress through uncertainty and the unknown, making life more interesting and enjoyable. These patterns grow into concepts, which are higher mental thought, AND we begin to search for a higher level of truth!

I guess that's worth an example. Hmmm. Perhaps a simple one. You're building a dollhouse for your daughter, and you've got everything figured out. She got a new doll for her birthday and Christmas is right around the corner, so you go at it. You've done this before, something simpler when she was younger, so you've got the know-how. And you do a beautiful job! You even build small pieces of furniture that are perfectly scaled to the house!

Christmas morning your daughter comes bounding down the steps with her birthday doll—who sleeps with her every night—lovingly under her arm. It is in that moment that you realize the doll is three inches taller than the height of the dollhouse room ceilings! While doll height was an input variable assumed from a past experience, now you have discovered a higher truth (pardon the play on words). First, that, like people, dolls come in various sizes and therefore have varying housing needs. Second, *there's a need for you to pay more attention to the small details of life that matter most to those who matter most to you*. Third, … well, you get the point.

Sustainability in the co-evolving state of this phase requires *empathy*, which provides a direct understanding of another individual, and a heightened awareness of the context of their lives, and their desires and needs in the moment at hand. In this phase we are clearly developing higher mental faculties and instinctive knowledge of the workings of the larger Universe, which helps cultivate intuition and develop insights in service to our self, our family and society.

As we recognize ever higher truths, we begin to see the connections among all things. A feeling of "Oneness" is emerging. For example, we recognize our relationship with the Earth, and that we are all part of a larger ecosystem. This recognition brings with it a deeper caring for the environment in which we live.

It is then that we enter **Phase 3 of the ISCJ**. As we expand and connect, we are able to tap into the larger intuitional field that energetically connects all people This can only be accomplished when energy is focused outward in service to the larger whole, requiring a deeper connection to others. Compassion deepens that connection.

In the progression of learning to navigate life represented by the three phases of this journey, we empower ourselves, developing our personal strengths and expanding our conscious awareness of who we are and how we relate to the world. Immersed in the human experience, we join in a neuronal dance with the Universe, with each of us in the driver's seat selecting our partners and directing our dance steps.

We'll further explore this movement from sympathy to empathy to compassion and beyond— all part of the ISCJ—in the last idea presented in this book.

[Your Thoughts]

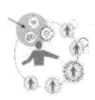

Idea 2: These times call for a Global Ethic.

As we prepared to enter the new century, the Assembly of Religious and Spiritual Leaders signed a declaration, "Towards a Global Ethic."[5] For the first time, there were Universally-accepted norms of behavior and responsibility, an ethics for humanity. This Global Ethic is *a call for humanity to live a more mature expression of moral life through the transformation of consciousness*.

This call, never more needed than in the changing, uncertain and complex environment of today, is not just to those who profess specific beliefs or practice specific religions. It is a larger call to humanity, and it is reverberating right above our upper threshold of awareness. Speaking poetically— or as my dad used to say, waxing eloquent—*with a soft push upwards, and the slightest widening of the eyes and opening of the heart, we can embrace this expression*.

This idea of "Universality" can be a tricky one. It doesn't mean everyone has to believe, think and value the same stuff ... that would be impossible. Nor would it be desirable! And there are plenty really good minds who believe that all existing things are particulars![6]

Now, a belief in the "absolute" would have a great deal more to do with faith than knowledge, which you may or may not have experienced. And, admittedly, the idea of a "Universal" is very close to the idea of an "absolute." The way we look at *Universals* is as having similarities of identity in terms of conditions, properties and relations. This means that Universals are higher-order patterns that have relationships that hold true *between other* Universals. Okay. As we learn more and more, maybe we just might be able to perceive something that's higher than these higher-order patterns! But, for now, a Universal, by definition, represents the highest order we can perceive in our still-growing-but-limited minds.

Wasn't that fun? Words and concepts can be really interesting and, if you followed all that and disagree, that's fun, too! Diversity is wonderful, and we can learn so much from each other since we each have different ways of thinking.

So, what is the advantage of thinking about a Global Ethic in terms of "Universal norms of behavior"? Well, a Universal spirituality would potentially provide direction for moving ahead with an undergirding of moral fabric. With some of the stuff that coming into our reality today, that would certainly e a good thing! Sir John Templeton, a financial investor and philanthropist, put it this way,

"Universal principles are like compasses; they always point the way."[7]

This idea of Universal norms of behavior is similar to the quality standards we develop for specific business products; for example, the American National Standard ISO 9000. The expectation of certain standards enables purchasers to trust the product, to know what they are getting. In like manner, there are certainly common standards that can be defined for living a moral life, practices that would support the transformation of consciousness.

In that assembly we talked about at the beginning of this idea, the group of spiritual leaders who participated came up with eight elements perceived as "essential" to a Universal spirituality. These are:

(1) An actualized moral capacity and commitment;
(2) Deep nonviolence and reverence for all life;
(3) A sense of interdependence and spiritual solidarity;
(4) Spiritual practice;
(5) Mature self-knowledge;
(6) Simplicity of life;
(7) Compassion and selfless service; and
(8) A witness to justice.

That's a pretty good set. Would you add anything?

Spiritual energy weaves itself throughout the physical, mental and emotional fields in which we all exist. *Spiritual* doesn't mean religion, which is the way we may or may not choose to practice our spiritual nature. We describe spirituality as *standing in relationship with others pertaining to matters of the soul*. Of course, that description requires us to define "soul."

Soul represents the animating principle of human life in terms of *thought and action*, specifically focused on its *moral aspects*, the *emotional part of human nature*, and *higher development of the mental faculties*. When we use this definition to look at the eight elements of a Universal spirituality listed above, we discover that (1) and (2) are primarily focused on moral aspects; (3) and (5) are primarily focused on higher development of the mental faculties; (1), (4), (6) and (8) are focused on actualized experiences—that's putting our spiritual nature into effective action; and (7) (which is *compassion and selfless service*) is focused on both the emotional part of human nature *and* putting our spiritual nature into effective action!

This validates our earlier thinking, so we must have been on track, and it represents an important characteristic of compassion. Yes, compassion is a state of being connected to morality and focused on the emotional part of human nature, yet it is also inclusive of a state of acting, *giving selfless service*!

The philosopher and educator John Beversluis, who writes about the need for a Global Ethic for Universal spirituality, feels that the transformation of an individual living an intense inner life leads to spontaneous development of a sensitivity to other's needs. This is when a person becomes capable of thinking and acting beyond his or her own self-interest, with the ability to figure out the needs of others, what they require. John says that this pattern of behavior "is found in every valid expression of the spiritual life and is one of the infallible signs of its genuineness."[8]

Let's see how we stack up with those characteristics that make up Universal Spirituality.

* * * * *

EXERCISE: *Tapping into a Universal Spirituality*

STEP 1: Take a moment to go back and review the eight elements perceived as "essential" to a Universal spirituality. Then, set those aside and reflect on your life.

STEP 2: Ask the following questions to yourself and reflect on your answers:

What actions do I take that show my moral capacity and commitment?

Do I have any violent tendencies? How do I handle these?

How do I treat others? How do I treat animals?

Do I feel like I'm part of a larger team? Do I feel a connection with others around the world? What are the connections among people and how do these connections play out in my life?

What spiritual practices do I participate in during my day-to-day life?

How well do I know myself? Am I a victim of life or do I choose the direction of my life?

Do I make things more complicated than they need to be? Do I enjoy the little things in life?

What are the things that I am compassionate about? When I feel compassion, how do I act on it?

Am I able to engage humility in interactions with others?

What is the relationship of justice to my beliefs and values? Do I see equal justice for all world citizens?

STEP 3: For any responses where you felt "uncomfortable" with your thoughts, make a note about that "feeling" and reflect on any changes you may wish to make to improve that "feeling."

STEP 4: MAKE THOSE CHANGES.

* * * * *

Idea 3: Empathy developed while co-evolving is a stepping stone toward conscious compassion.

During the linear cause-and-effect phase of the Intelligent Social Change Journey (ISCJ) introduced in our first idea, sympathy is required. We've all felt sympathy for someone else. You care about someone, are sorry for their troubles, and want to support them. And this caring about others can help reduce forces, making it easier to have successful outcomes in difficult situations. For example, if you have a responsible employee that is working furiously to keep up a heavy workload while simultaneously trying to support a seriously ill spouse, you might offer a home work option that provides a win-win solution.

As we move into the co-evolving phase of our developmental journey, a deeper connection to others is necessary. This deeper connection is empathy.

Both sympathy and empathy have Greek roots in the term *pathos*, which means feeling or suffering. Empathy is the entanglement of intuition, resonance and sympathy, simultaneously processed through physical, mental and emotional channels. This combination is an objective attempt to try and live the inner life of another person.

A good starting point to developing empathy is to develop a good understanding of your *self*, including your physical and mental capabilities and your emotional guidance system. Without this understanding, the boundaries between self and others can easily blur, such that the inner states of others are assumed to be identical with your inner states. This fusion prevents an objective perspective and leads to confusion in relationships and difficulties in co-evolving. People are not the same.

Empathy can be thought of in three different ways. First, as *perspective-taking*, seeing the world through someone else's eyes. Second, some people can literally feel another person's emotions, which causes a *personal distress*. Third, the ability to recognize another's emotional state and tune into it, developing an *empathic concern*.[9] All three of these types of empathy provide a direct understanding of another individual, a heightened awareness of the context of their lives, as well as awareness of their desires and needs in the moment at hand.

Interestingly, the physiological basis for empathy is so inherent in brain function that it has been extensively documented in other primates. For example, in a study of rhesus monkeys, when one monkey pulled a chain for food a shock was given to that monkey's companion. The monkey who pulled the chain refused to pull it again for 12 days, that is, the primates would literally choose to starve themselves rather than inflict pain on their companions![10] As Dutch primatologist Frans de Waal observed: *Empathy is nature's lesson for a kinder society.*[11]

A key component of empathy is feeling, and there are findings from neuroscience that suggest that through feelings there is an active link between *our own* bodies and minds and the bodies and minds of *those around us*. What happens is that the insula cortex and anterior cingulate in the brain actually become activated either *when we experience pain*, **or** *when a loved one experiences pain*! And the degree of activation of these two structures has been shown to correlate with measures of empathy.[12]

I bet if you think back a bit, you'll remember a time when you felt another person's pain, or when you were fully engaged in another person's joy. That's empathy. And as these experiences increase, you begin to recognize the similarities among people—the highs, the lows, the joy, the sadness, all happening at different times—and, if you choose, with this awareness, you've begun the journey into conscious compassion.

Developing Conscious Compassion

Perhaps the best way to fully understand conscious compassion is to conceptually merge the concepts of "conscious" and "compassion." So first, let's look at descriptive definitions that have come up during our discussion side-by-side.

Conscious	Compassion
•A state of awareness •A private, selective and continuous change process •A sequential set of ideas, thoughts images, feelings and perceptions •An understanding of the connections and relationship among them and or self	•A sympathy for the trouble/suffering of others, often including a desire to help •A state of being connected to morality and focused on the emotional part of human nature •Inclusive of a state of acting, giving selfless service •Includes sympathy: the feeling that you care about and are sorry about someone else's trouble; a feeling of support for something or someone •Includes empathy: the capacity to put oneself in the shoes of another, to understand and even experience the emotions ideas, beliefs and opinions of another

Table 1. *Descriptive definitions of "conscious" and "compassion."*

Okay. Second, merging these descriptive definitions, we get these bullet points:

- Active awareness and understanding of others' thoughts and feelings as situations present themselves in the context of life.
- A moral responsibility and desire to intelligently and wisely care for and support others.

- Recognition and understanding of the connections and relationships among people and events, and the potential outcomes of actions taken.
- A conscious choice to give selfless service.

Now comes the trick part, putting it all together. By exploring these multiple descriptive definitions, we can now define conscious compassion as *an intelligent choice to give selfless service based on active awareness and understanding of others thoughts and feelings, the relationships among people and events, and wisdom.*

This does not insinuate a separation from emotions, but rather the intelligence and wisdom of an individual who has embraced emotions and feelings as an integral part of life, using them as a guidance system and fuel to intelligently and wisely act.

[Your Thoughts]

Idea 4: The act of judging can derail compassion.

The innate ability to evoke meaning through understanding and comprehension—to evaluate, judge and decide—distinguishes the human mind from most other life forms. To judge is the act of forming an opinion, interpretation or conclusion. The ability to judge enables us to discriminate and discern—to see similarities and differences, comprehend and form patterns from particulars, and purposefully create, store and apply knowledge.

There is an element of judging in every decision we make. For example, building up expertise in an area of knowledge requires (1) feedback on decisions and actions, (2) active engagement in getting and interpreting this feedback, that is, judging its value, not passively allowing someone else to do so, and (3) repetitions, which provide the opportunity to practice making decisions and getting feedback.[13]

While not necessarily widely recognized, judgments are used far more than logic or rational thinking in making decisions. This is because all but the simplest decisions occur in a context in which there is insufficient, noisy, or *perhaps too much information* to make rational conclusions.

Think back to the last time you made an important decision. Be honest, now. What was that decision based on? Was it fully driven by a logic trail? What you may have realized already is that judging is very much connected with emotional context related to preferences, that is, what you like or don't like.

Understanding that judging serves as a valuable human tool for operating in this world, in relation to compassion we move the focus of this discussion to the judging of others. **Judging others is the opposite of compassion.**

The *act* of judging others and their actions requires something or someone to judge against. When one person is judging another person, it is in the context of a scale, with the person who is judging generally located somewhere in the middle of that scale. If the person who is judging is egotistical, arrogant or insecure with himself, there may be a need to judge others as less in order to prove personal superiority or (artificially) feel better about himself.

Alternately, if a person's self-regard is low, she may judge others above herself, which will prove or justify her feelings and add to her insecurity. Thus, as Wayne Dyer so succinctly said, "When you judge others, you do not define them; you define yourself."[14]

Often, the people we are judging are showing us *a part of ourselves that we do not like*, or that they are comfortable with things we are unable to do. For example,

"We may judge a busty lady for wearing a tight shirt that emphasizes her bosom for dressing cheap, when we are jealous of her physique or her courage to dress as she pleases. We may judge a working mom for not staying at home with her kids when we are a housewife who always dreamt of a career but gave it up when she became pregnant. We may judge a couple kissing openly in the streets because we dream of being in love, but are too afraid to open our heart for someone."[15]

The act of gossip may accompany the act of judging. We've all experienced gossiping in some way, whether we participated in it, or just overheard it. Gossip is the sharing of negative opinions in order to justify those negative opinions or justify self. Again, gossip is more about the individual who is gossiping than the subject of that gossip.

<<<<<<<>>>>>>

INSIGHT: **Similar to judging, gossip, the sharing of negative opinions in order to justify those opinions or self, is more about the individual who is gossiping than the subject of that gossip.**

<<<<<<<>>>>>>

When we get into patterns of judging and gossiping, it may be difficult to catch ourselves in the act, and when we are in the company of others who do so, it is easy for similar behaviors to creep into habit. The short tool "Discerning Judging" can help.

* * * * *

EXERCISE: *Discerning Judging*

Remember, change begins with awareness, and only you can change yourself. This exercise is focused on exploring negative thoughts and feelings that occurred in the past about an individual, and how those differ from thoughts and feelings you have about that same individual today. This exercise will only work if you are forthright and honest.

STEP 1: Find a place where you can be comfortable and uninterrupted. Have a pad of paper and pen in front of you.

STEP 2: Write down the names of people with whom you have had a conflict or about whom you have had negative feelings IN THE PAST. Indicate an approximate date of conflict or negative event. Leave a couple of lines of space after each name.

STEP 3: Starting at the top of the list, one-by-one, think about the event that triggered the conflict or negative feelings. Imagine yourself back in that event, and quickly jot down FROM THAT VIEWPOINT the thoughts and feelings about that person you are experiencing. Be honest. You can trigger your memory by thinking about the location, details leading up to that event, and your personal responses to that event.

STEP 4: When you are done, put that list aside and forget it for 15-20 minutes. Purposefully focus your attention on something positive and of interest IN THE NOW. Get up and have a drink of water and a snack, something that you like to eat.

STEP 5: Now, go back to your list, and, still feeling good and with a good taste in your mouth, from this new frame of reference review each name and what you have written, asking: Is this judging (criticism) or is this discerning (perceiving)? Mark a "J" or a "P" beside each descriptive phrase.

STEP 6: For each place you have marked a "J," now describe this person from your current frame of reference.

Repeat this exercise as needed.

* * * * *

More about discernment. Discernment is to make out clearly, to perceive or recognize difference. One more time, we defer to the wisdom of the financial investor and philanthropist, Sir John Templeton, to help us understand this concept. "Discernment can help us comprehend where another person is on his or her path of growth and eliminate any need to be upset because he or she may come from a different place. Discernment perceives; judgment criticizes."[16]

<<<<<<<◇>>>>>>>

INSIGHT: **Discernment perceives; judgment criticizes.**

<<<<<<<◇>>>>>>>

Judging is a capacity that carries with it a large responsibility associated with how it is used. As we mature and learn who we are, the judging of others gives way to awareness and discernment. We have developed a knowing of who we are. In our interactions it is no longer necessary to contrast others on our personal scale. The level of awareness and trust of others, of course, is dependent on the relationship in which you have chosen to engage.

As judgment turns to awareness, enabling discernment and discretion without judgment, compassion grows.

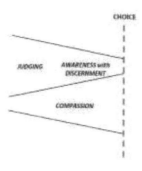

Figure 2. *As judging grows to awareness with discernment, compassion grows.*

We are now developing an understanding of the other without constructing any forces with respect to our own inner feelings or shortcomings. We no longer are holding up the measurement scale with ourselves in the middle of that scale. Rather, we are learning to honor, and have compassion for, diversity and choice of both ourselves and others.

[Your Thoughts]

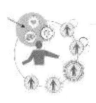

Idea 5: Compassion cannot be achieved when we retain strong negative emotions.

Sometimes when we are caught in the middle of a situation where strong emotions have been embedded, it is difficult to move beyond that place, and it may still be difficult years after the event is long past! This is because emotional tags, regardless of whether they are negative or positive, create strong connections among the neurons of our brain.

When we are caught up in our own emotions, there is little room to consider others. Imagine newlyweds who are oblivious to the crowd around them! Or, think about the last time you were really angry. When negative emotions such as anger take over, it is easy to become enraged and filled with hatred. These emotions are destructive and can wind up causing both short and long-term damage.

The Dalai Lama reminds us that we should act on the world with calm and clarity. I hear one of you asking, "Who is the Dalai Lama?" The short answer is that he is the spiritual leader of Tibet, although the current Dalai Lama is also the political leader of the government in exile. A Tibetan Buddhist, he is believed to be the 14th incarnation of the Buddha of Compassion. He certainly models that title in his words and actions.

The Dalai Lama believes in what he calls *Universal compassion*, emphasizing that there is a distinction between the act, which is unacceptable, and the actor, within whom is the potential for change. In other words, having compassion for someone does not mean that you are *approving* of their decisions and actions in a situation, but rather that you see the goodness in the person, have an appreciation of the situation they find themselves in, and see their potential for change.

<<<<<<<◇>>>>>>

INSIGHT: **There is a distinction between the act, which is unacceptable, and the actor, within whom is the potential for change.**

<<<<<<<◇>>>>>>

The Dalai Lama also says that Universal compassion is a hard goal to achieve. As he contends, it is difficult to go up against the natural inclination to favor our own group—our family, company or ethnic group. "So, the first step is to overcome that tendency and to become more accepting of and caring toward a wider circle of people."[17]

The final step is caring for everyone, achieving a Universal compassion. Again, we see a call to action as the Dalai Lama voices, *Don't just talk about it, do something*.[18]

Idea 6: Conscious compassion is an intelligent choice to give selfless service.

It's strange having a question repeatedly overtake the monkey chatter in our mind about an event that occurred 34 years ago! Well, that's exactly what's happening.

Thirty-four years ago, I was living in Yokosuka, Japan, on the U.S. Naval Base. This was an amazing time of life ... I'd always wanted to live abroad, and the Japanese lifestyle and ceremony of life provided not only a rich taste of that dream, but oh so many learning experiences!

The day after arriving on Base, I was out hunting for a job, and within the week was hired as a part-time writer for the *Seahawk*, the Base weekly newspaper. There were over 40,000 military personnel and families living on and off the Base, and with the ships often out to sea, you can imagine the need to have support systems for those waiting for the Fleet to return.

There were lots of opportunities to make a difference. Since I'd had an early career in music, one of those ways was leading the various choirs through the all-Faith Chapel of Hope. Another was participating in some way in musicals. Another was manning the help hotline on Friday and Saturday nights. And another was through writing about the many discoveries available to all of us on and off Base. So, I did.

Pretty soon, that job was full-time, then, it was as the editor of the paper, expanding to include working with *Pacific Stars and Stripes* every week and writing columns for the English paper, *Tokyo Weekender*. I never knew what adventure was next!

Then, near the middle of November in 1984, I received a phone call that caused this little book to be such an important part of my life. For the first time in *her* life—and maybe the only time—Mother Teresa agreed to visit a military base.[19] She had spoken earlier at the International School in Tokyo, then visited a hospital in Hamamatsu. And from there, a U.S. Army C-12 flew her to Atsugi from where she was heloed to Camp Zama.

Mother was greeted by the Senior Chaplain of Camp Zama Chapel and a group of people who had worked with her mission in Tokyo. The Chaplain voiced all of our thoughts: "I can't say it's a once-in-a-lifetime experience because most people don't have it happen in their lifetime. It was one of those things that happen and I'm just happy to be a part of it." Together, the group joined in a meal of chicken, baked beans, bread and Indian tea with sugar and cream.

Then it was my turn. With Father Andre Gogaert sitting next to her on a sofa and me a couple of feet away on a facing chair, we spoke. She leaned towards me, perhaps a product of the bent form, and tilted her leathery face upward so that her eyes could take in my face, could follow my expression. Her mouth was slightly, knowingly, curled upward at the edges, laughing at the moment, and her eyes … and her eyes … I don't have the words.

She began in English, greeting me, asking after me, two old friends in a sweet embrace of caring. And then she would listen carefully as I asked questions, looking aside to Father Andre when she needed clarification, which was provided in French! And, that's the question that keeps popping up in my head: Why French?

Mother was born in 1910 in what is now Yugoslavia, and by the age of 18 had joined a group of Irish nuns in the Archdiocese of Calcutta, and then called to serve, to bring aid and dignity to the destitute in her adopted country of India. So why French? But perhaps that question interrupts the flow of the story.

On the other hand, did the story really begin in 1984? I think not. While I remember hearing about then-Sister Teresa on and off in my early years, this story began ten years earlier following a musical performance on a New York stage. Two little, old women (who were about my age now … but, alas, then I thought they were old!) came running backstage to get an autograph. Quite eloquently, I smiled and answered, "Of course!"

Taking hold of the program and a pen offered my way, my hand paused above the program. I couldn't remember my name! *Who was I?* Gosh, I'd played so many roles in my life, both on and off-stage. From the life stories people have shared with us when visiting the Mountain Quest Inn here in the Allegheny Mountains of West Virginia, I'm pretty sure *most* of us are living shifting lives full of lots of varied learning experiences!

Back home, reflecting on this event throughout the evening, I decided if I didn't know who I was, then I could CHOOSE who I am and who I wanted to be. So, I called to mind those people who I deeply admired and appreciated—my father, my mentor and Sister Teresa—and asked myself, ***Why*** *do I feel this way about them? While I can't be them, what traits do they exhibit that I can learn from and make my own?*

And there is the crux of this story. From Sister Teresa, I desired to learn persistence and *compassion*. Now, ten years later, in her presence, I could *feel* her compassion as she answered my questions, sometimes in English, and sometimes in French, which was translated by Father Andre.

"At the age of twelve I first knew I had a vocation to help the poor" she shared. This was consistent with what I had read about her. It was in her eighteenth year that she left to join the Sisters of Loretto. She took her first vows as a nun in 1928, and her final vows nine years later.

During her work of teaching and serving as principal at St. Mary's High School in Calcutta, her heart was greatly touched by the suffering children, lepers, and destitute ill outside the cloister walls. In 1946—the year before I was born—she received what she called a *call within a call*. "The message was clear." Her eyes sparkled as she said these words, and it was clear to me where that message came from! There was a small cross, anchored to her head wrap with a safety pen at the side of her head, that slightly fluttered as she moved her head to motion the Father to translate. She continued, "I was to leave the convent and help the poor, while living among them." This call came in 1948 at which time Mother Teresa founded the Society of the Missionaries of Charity in Calcutta's slums.

Now, these kinds of words have been written about her, maybe even the same words, since no doubt she had memorized them in English, but as she said them to me, they came from the wholeness of who she was. Now, *I* was leaning towards *her* and, occasionally in a gesture, an accent to a shared thought, we touched. Did we sit there talking an hour or two? I do not know how long it was.

When she went into the Camp Zama gymnasium to speak, twelve hundred expectant faces awaited her appearance. She did not disappoint. The 73-year-old, slight form entered the side door, paused to exchange smiles with a young child, and, with back bowed and hands clasped in front of her, edged gracefully up the stairs onto the platform, aided by Father Andre. I followed with her.

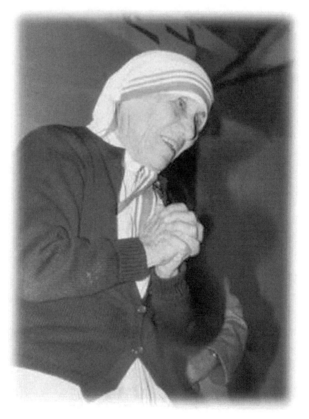

Figure 2. *She did not disappoint. With hands clasped and a smile on her face, she welcomed the crowd.*

Mother Teresa spoke. Softly. Vibrantly. Her message was one of love, repeating the good news brought to this world, that "He loves the world. That He loves you and He loves me and He loves that leper …"

She shared stories filled with compassion, and to this group she spoke in clear English. "A few weeks ago, two young people came to our house. They gave me lots of money and I asked them where do you get so much money? They said two days ago we got married and before we married we decided to have no wedding feast. To have no wedding clothes. To give the money to you to feed the people, your people. I was surprised and asked them about it. They answered, 'We wanted to share the joy of love by giving' …

"Hunger is not for bread alone. Hunger is for love …

"I will never forget one day walking down a street in London. I saw a man sitting looking very lonely, so I went right up to him. I reached for his hands. They were so cold. He looked up at me and said, 'After such a long time I'm feeling the warmth of a human hand.' And he had a smile on his face because there was someone who loved him …

"Small things are special to us … today people are so terribly busy that they have no time to even smile at each other … God speaks in the silence of the heart …

**"The world has never needed peace so much
as today. Where will the peace begin? …**

There was more. I regret not having my notes
at hand. She asked the question so quietly, yet so
poignantly, capturing the hearts of all those who
leaned toward her to hear every word. Reflecting,
this question has haunted me for many years. We
look at our world today, and still we ask it. Where
will the peace begin?

Mother lowered her head, then with a soft
smile began, "A few days before I came here a poor
man came to our house, a poor man from the slums,
and he said his only child was dying and the doctor
had prescribed this special medicine that could be
gotten only from England. I said I would do what I
could. He gave me the prescription. Just at that
moment a man came in with a basket of medicine.
We have people that we send to families and they
gather the leftover medicine from the people of
Calcutta. This man came with the basket of half-used
medicine and what was on the top of all the
medicines—*that* medicine, the one that the doctor
had prescribed.

"Had he come before, had he come after, I
would not have seen him. But he came just at that
moment.

"Out of the millions and millions and millions
of children in the world, God was concerned for that

little boy in Calcutta. God's concern for us is so great …

"I will pray for you, for your families, for the work *you* have to do. **I will pray for you that you grow in holiness. For holiness is not the luxury of the few. It is the simple duty for every one of us.**"

There were twelve hundred people pushing (gently) to reach her hand. Others, who had already done so, struggled to retreat through the crowd, faces glowing with love.

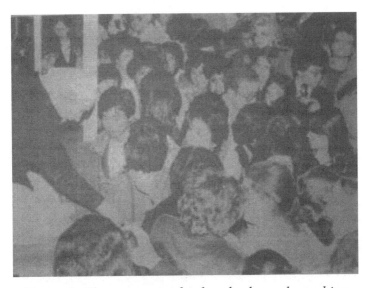

Figure 3. *There were twelve hundred people pushing (gently) to reach her hand.*

I circled down the stairs to get some photo shots from in front of her. It was nearly an impossible task to accomplish: heads and hands bobbed constantly in and out of the field. Then, I was right there in front of her. A young girl beside me reached out to Mother and pressed Mother's hand against her cheek. Then, those sparkling dark eyes in their small earth-worn frame turned to me. Again.

The twelve hundred disappeared. My hand reached towards hers; the camera dropped to the length of its neck strap. Her grasp was firm and carried with it a warmth that tingled my knuckles and spread rapidly up my forearm.

Our locked eyes reached beyond the soft pushing and struggling of the moment, and continued into our very souls. I do not know what she found; I discovered a love so deep, a giving so great, a compassion so …

Again, words fail me. For 40 years now, I've sought to learn that compassion, to make it mine, but the lesson is never done. There are always new situations emerging, new circumstances, as each and every one of us is tossed into the challenges of life. For example, when dementia becomes the bedfellow of a loved one, and the trials of life must be addressed through this lens.

And so, in this state of growth, I defer to my poet laureate, Cindy Lee Scott to give me the words:

Growth

Soul touch

Love so deep

Giving so great

Compassion so vast

Selflessness so complete

Immersed in the light of Truth

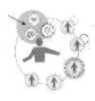

Idea 7: Compassion is part of the larger journey toward unconditional love.

The words and actions of Mother Teresa enabled us to see her selflessness and *feel* her compassion, and through her life choices we recognized her persistence in following this path, her call within a call. And for Mother Teresa, we know this persistence came from a place of deep love.

The expansion from sympathy to empathy to compassion is part of a larger continuum based on an increasing depth of connection, which is developing an inner sense focused in the heart energy center. As we move up the continuum toward unconditional love, there is an increased balancing of senses across the physical, mental and emotional parts of who we are.

There is a direct correlation between this continuum and the phase changes of the Intelligent Social Change Journey introduced in Idea 1 in this book. This means that as we move from linear cause and effect to co-evolving with our environment, it is necessary to deepen our understanding of others, moving from sympathy to empathy. And as we move towards recognition of the larger ecosystem of which we are a part and opening to energies of that intuitional plane, that ever-deepening connection emerges as compassion. And it is through compassion that we begin to touch agápē love.

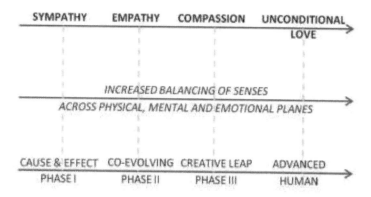

Figure 4. *From sympathy to unconditional love: a continuum with an increasing depth of connection.*

The movement from sympathy to empathy to compassion to unconditional love can be slowed or stopped through compassion fatigue, a loss or loosening of sympathy for the misfortune of others because too many demands have been made on the feelings of an individual. This is an *overwhelment* that can harden the heart. An example is the actions of some military members during World War II, and, more recently, interrogators engaged in military prisons, whose belief sets did not support their actions.

This did not happen to Mother Teresa. Even when she entered what she described as "the dark night of the soul" she did not lose her faith and her persistence in her call within a call did not falter. The extraordinary set of actions that created the pattern of her life serve as an example for us all.

My emotions are running deep as I recall these special moments of my life. Emotions are a building block of consciousness. Indeed, we live "within a sea of experienced and expressed emotions."[20] Reflect on a past experience where your emotions have taken over your thoughts, and perhaps your actions. We have all had this experience, which helps us to recognize just how powerful our emotional system can be!

There is a constant interplay of the physical and mental with the emotional going on throughout the body. In fact, Candice Pert, a neuroscientist and pharmacologist, discovered that there are actually information-processing receptors on most of the body's cells.[21] This means that signals are sent throughout the body as part of a single intelligent system. The "mind" is not focused in the head, but throughout the body!

Love first develops through consciousness, generally related by a growing child to the parent or caregiver. Later the concept takes on different meanings, and during puberty this feeling of strong affection becomes attached to the idea of romance and sexual desire.

This strong affection also accompanies developing beliefs; for example, a growing connection to God. The highest form of this love— the love of God for man, and the love of man for God—is called agápē. This Universal, unconditional love that transcends all things is derived from the ancient Greek, ἀγάπη, agápē, which translates as gaping the mouth wide open, as with wonder and expectation.[22]

Love is a powerful force. Viktor Frankl, who endured three years at Auschwitz and other Nazi prisons, discovered the power of love in the midst of his suffering. The realization came as an image of his wife vividly arose in his mind. His words are so very powerful that, if you will excuse me, I'd very much like to share his exact words with you! I think it would be okay with him, so here goes:

"A thought transfixed me: for the first time in my life I saw the truth as it is set into song by so many poets, proclaimed as the final wisdom by so many thinkers. **The truth—that love is the ultimate and the highest goal to which man can aspire.** Then I grasped the meaning of the greatest secret that human poetry and human thought and belief have to impart: *The salvation of man is through love and in love.* I understood how a man who has nothing left in this world still may know bliss, be it only for a brief moment, in the contemplation of his beloved. In a position of utter desolation, when many cannot express himself in positive action, when his only achievement may consist in enduring his sufferings in the right way—an honorable way—in such a position man can, through loving contemplation of the image he carries of his beloved, achieve fulfillment. For the first time in my life I was able to understand the meaning of the words, 'The angels are lost in perpetual contemplation of an infinite glory'."[23]

Again and again, Frankl was able to find his way back from the prisoner's existence to this place of love. He did not know whether his wife was alive or not, but he did know one thing, that "Love goes very far beyond the physical person of the beloved. It finds its deepest meaning in his spiritual being, his inner self. Whether or not he is actually present, whether or not he is still at all, ceases somehow to be of importance." [24]

Love is born of understanding another, truly knowing another, looking within at their motives, sentiments and values. And once you really know who someone is, love is contagious, expanding when it is given away. Imagine the field becoming larger and larger, becoming a stream and connecting everyone to everyone. Is this possible? Can so much start from such small beginnings?

Just maybe we've already started this journey. As we recognize our connectedness to others there is a steady and continuous development of unconditional love. Agápē, this unconditional love, is an attribute of the advanced human, developed through "the acceptance and understanding of ALL things created in the Universe."[25] It emerges as we progress through the Intelligent Social Change Journey, expanding through sympathy to empathy, through empathy to compassion, and, ultimately, with wonder and expectation, through compassion reaching toward unconditional love.

What does this mean to me?

Bottom line time. This had some good sharing and it certainly makes good sense. But what is my take-away? How can all this make a difference in my experience of life, in my job, in my relationships?

Let's recall a few highlights, and you might reflect on how you might change your behaviors in response to each of these learnings.

- In order to co-evolve with the larger world, we need to develop a deeper understanding of ourselves and of others.

- The transformation of an individual living an intense inner life leads to spontaneous development of a sensitivity to other's needs.

- Empathy helps us to understand others; compassion moves us to act on that understanding.

- Often, the people we are judging are showing us a part of ourselves that we do not like.

- Strong negative emotions interfere with our ability to be compassionate toward others.

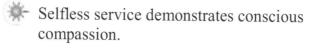 Selfless service demonstrates conscious compassion.

Love is contagious. It expands when it is given away.

Choose compassion.

YOU can make a difference in this world!

This volume of **Conscious Look Books** builds conversationally on the ideas presented in *The Profundity and Bifurcation of Change Parts I-V:* "Introduction to the Intelligent Social Change Journey"; *Part IV: Learning from the Past*, largely presented in Chapter 35: "Conscious Compassion" and *Part III: Learning in the Present*, Chapter 19, "Emotions as a Guidance System," and Chapter 20, "Stuck Energy: Limiting and Accelerating." Co-authors of the original text include David Bennet, Arthur Shelley, Theresa Bullard, John Lewis and Donna Panucci. Full references are available in the original text, which is published by MQIPress, Frost, WV (2017), and available as an eBook on www.amazon.com

Endnotes

[1] *American Heritage Dictionary of the English Language* (4th ed.) (2006). Boston: Houghton Mifflin Company, 585.

[2] See Damasio, A.R. (1999). *Descartes' error: Emotion, Reason, and the Human Brain*. New York: G.P. Putnam's Sons. "The term feeling should be reserved for the private, mental experience of an emotion, while the term emotion should be used to designate the collection of responses, many of which are publicly observable," 42.

[3] Quoted from Lerner, M. (2000). *Spirit Matters*. Charlottesville, VA: Hampton Roads.

[4] Intelligent activity is a state of interaction where intent, purpose, direction, values and expected outcomes are clearly understood and communicated among all parties, reflecting wisdom and achieving a higher truth.

[5] See Beversluis, J. (Ed.) (1993). "The Declaration of a Global Ethic," signed by 143 respected leaders from the world's major faiths at the 1993 Parliament of the World's Religions held in Chicago, IL on September 4, 1993. Retrieved 11/20/16 from http://www.religioustolerance.org/parliame.htm

[6] See Locke, J. (2016). *Essay Concerning Human Understanding*, Book III, p. 377. Retrieved 10/23/16 from http://mypages.iit.edu/~schmaus/Origins_of_Modern_Philosophy/lectures/Locke.htm

[7] Quoted from Templeton, J. (2002). *Wisdom from World Religions: Pathways Toward Heaven on Earth.* Philadelphia, PA: Templeton Foundation Press, 257.

[8] Quoted from Beversluis, J. (2000). *Cross-Examining Socrates: A Defense of the Interlocutors in Plato's Early Dialogues.* Cambridge: Cambridge University Press, 243.

[9] See Riggio, R.E. (2015). "Are You Empathic? 3 Types of Empathy and What They Mean." Retrieved 09/14/15 from https://www.psychologytoday.com/blog/cutting-edge-leadership/201108/are-you-empathic-3-types-empathy-and-what-they-mean

[10] See Masserman, J., Wechkin, M.S. and Terris, W. (1964). "Altruistic Behavior in Rhesus Monkeys" in *Am. J. Psychiatry 121*, 584-85.

[11] See de Waal, F. (2009). *The Age of Empathy: Nature's Lessons for a Kinder Society.* New York: Harmony Books.

[12] See Cozolino, L.J. (2006). *The Neuroscience of Human Relationships: Attachment and the Developing Social Brain.* New York: W.W. Norton.

[13] See Klein, G. (2003). *Intuition at Work: Why Developing Your Gut Instincts Will Make You Better at What You Do.* New York: Doubleday.

[14] Quoted from Templeton, 240.

[15] Quoted from Wilrieke (2016). "Judging Others Is About You" from Pure Wilrieke web log. Retrieved 09/30/16 from http://www.purewilrieke.com/judging-others-is-about-you

[16] Quoted from Templeton, p. 240.

[17] See Suttie, J. (2015), "Can Compassion Change the World" (Interview of Daniel Goleman re his book *A Force for Good: The Dalai Lama's Vision for Our World*). Retrieved 101716 from http://grreatergood.berkeley.edu/article/item/can_compassion_change_the_world

[18] See D. Goleman (2015), *A Force for Good: The Dalai Lama's Vision for Our World*, New York: Bantam Books.

[19] The author (then Alex Dean) wrote an article that detailed this visit which appeared in the November 30, 1984, *Seahawk* Vol. XXXV, No. 48, U.S. Fleet Activities, Yokosuka, Japan. Over the next few weeks, this article was reprinted in U.S. Navy newspapers throughout the world. Also, included as an appendix in A. Bennet and D. Bennet (2010), *The Journey into the Myst*, Frost, WV: MQIPress. Portions of this article are included in this text.

[20] Quoted from H. Plotkin (1994), *Darwin Machines and the Nature of Knowledge*, Cambridge, MA: Harvard University Press, 211.

[21] C.B. Pert (1997), *Molecules of Emotion: A Science Behind Mind-Body Medicine*, New York: Touchstone. As noted in B. Lipton (2005), *The Biology of Belief: Unleashing the Power of Consciousness*, Carlsbad, CA: Hay House, p. 132: This "established that the 'mind' was not focused in the head, but was distributed via signal molecules to the whole body."

[22] Merriam-Webster (2016). Retrieved 070616 http://www.webster-dictionary.org/definition/Agape

[23] Quoted from V.E. Frankl (1939/1963), *Man's Search for Meaning: an Introduction of Logotherapy*, New York: Pocket Books, 58-59.

[24] Ibid, p. 60.

[25] Cooper, L.R. (2005). *The Grand Vision: The Design and Purpose of a Human Being*. Ft. Collins, CO: Planetary Heart, 42.

The Volumes in
Possibilities that are YOU!

All Things in Balance

The Art of Thought Adjusting

Associative Patterning and Attracting

Beyond Action

Connections as Patterns

Conscious Compassion

The Creative Leap

The Emerging Self

The Emoting Guidance System

Engaging Forces

The ERC's of Intuition

Grounding

The Humanness of Humility

Intention and Attention

Knowing

Living Virtues for Today

ME as Co-Creator

Seeking Wisdom

Staying on the Path

Transcendent Beauty

Truth in Context

Made in the USA
Middletown, DE
25 June 2021